HEALTHY MACRO DIET MEAL PLANS

PLANS

Customizable and Delicious Recipes for Every Goal

Dr Lily Morgan

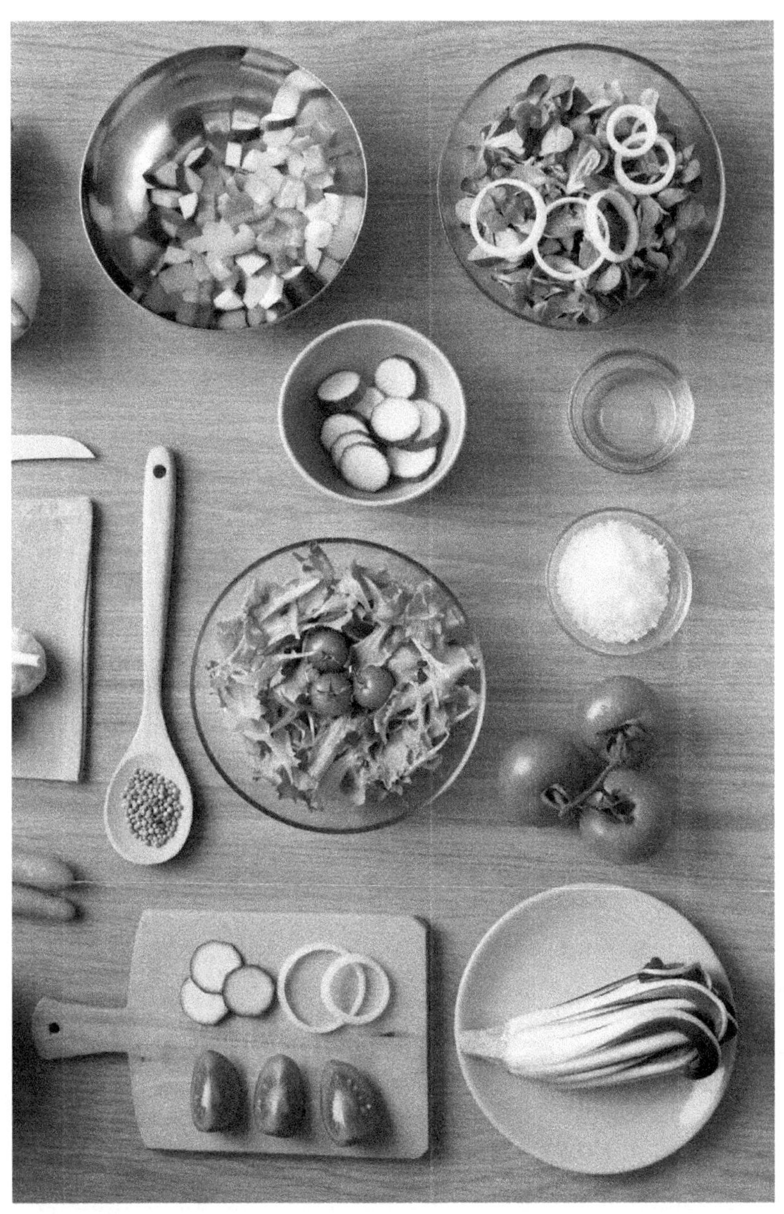

TABLE OF CONTENTS

Chapter 3: Lunch Recipes...................................... 36

Chapter 6: Desserts 81

INTRODUCTION

In today's fast-paced world, where countless diets and nutrition plans abound, the macro dieting approach stands out as a science-backed method for achieving and maintaining a healthier lifestyle. But why should you choose macro dieting, and what exactly are macronutrients?

Why Macro Dieting Matters

Macro dieting, also known as flexible dieting or IIFYM (If It Fits Your Macros), goes beyond simple calorie counting. It revolves around the idea that not all calories are created equal. Instead, it places a strong emphasis on the quality and composition of the calories you consume.

Unlike restrictive diets that eliminate entire food groups or demonize specific nutrients, macro dieting offers a balanced and sustainable approach. It recognizes that everyone's nutritional needs are unique and that achieving your fitness goals shouldn't mean giving up foods you love.

By adopting a macro-based approach, you gain a deeper understanding of your body's nutritional requirements. It empowers you to make informed choices about what you eat, helping you reach your goals while still enjoying a wide variety of foods. Whether your aim is to lose weight, gain muscle, or simply lead a healthier life, macro dieting provides a flexible framework to achieve your desired outcomes.

Cracking the Macronutrient Code

Now, let's dive into the core of macro dieting – macronutrients. These are the essential nutrients your body needs in relatively large quantities for optimal functioning. The three primary macronutrients are:

1. **Proteins**: Often referred to as the building blocks of life, proteins play a pivotal role in muscle repair, immune function, and the production of hormones and enzymes. They are commonly found in meat, poultry, fish, eggs, dairy products, and plant-based sources like beans and tofu.

2. **Carbohydrates**: Carbs are your body's primary source of energy. They come in various forms, including sugars, starches, and fiber. Whole grains, fruits, vegetables, and legumes are rich sources of carbohydrates that provide sustained energy and essential nutrients.

3. **Fats**: Dietary fats are crucial for overall health. They aid in the absorption of fat-soluble vitamins, support cell growth, and provide a backup source of energy. Healthy fats can be found in avocados, nuts, seeds, and fatty fish like salmon.

Understanding the role of these macronutrients is key to tailoring your diet to your specific needs. The macro dieting approach involves setting individualized macronutrient targets, allowing you to meet your fitness goals while enjoying a diverse and satisfying range of foods.

In this journey through macro dieting, you'll explore the art of balancing these macronutrients to create meals that nourish your body, boost your energy, and help you achieve the vibrant, healthy lifestyle you deserve. So, let's embark on this exciting path of discovery and empowerment as we delve deeper into the world of macro dieting and macronutrient mastery.

Chapter 1: 30 Day Meal Plan

Week 1:

Day 1:

- Breakfast: Protein-Packed Scrambled Eggs
- Lunch: Grilled Chicken Salad with Avocado
- Dinner: Baked Salmon with Lemon and Dill
- Snack: Greek Yogurt and Berries
- Dessert: Dark Chocolate Avocado Mousse

Day 2:

- Breakfast: Greek Yogurt Parfait with Berries
- Lunch: Quinoa and Black Bean Bowl
- Dinner: Grilled Turkey Burgers with Sweet Potato Fries
- Snack: Almonds and Dried Cranberries
- Dessert: Greek Yogurt Parfait with Honey

Day 3:

- Breakfast: Oatmeal with Almonds and Bananas
- Lunch: Tuna Salad Lettuce Wraps

- Dinner: Quinoa-Stuffed Bell Peppers

- Snack: Cottage Cheese with Pineapple

- Dessert: Berry Sorbet

Day 4:

- Breakfast: Spinach and Mushroom Omelette

- Lunch: Turkey and Veggie Stir-Fry

- Dinner: Spaghetti Squash with Turkey Meatballs

- Snack: Trail Mix with Nuts and Seeds

- Dessert: Protein-Packed Chocolate Brownies

Day 5:

- Breakfast: Chia Seed Pudding with Mango

- Lunch: Lentil Soup with Spinach

- Dinner: Teriyaki Tofu Stir-Fry

- Snack: Sliced Cucumber with Tzatziki

- Dessert: Chia Seed Pudding with Cocoa

Day 6:

- Breakfast: Avocado Toast with Poached Egg

- Lunch: Salmon with Asparagus

- Dinner: Chicken and Vegetable Skewers

- Snack: Edamame with Sea Salt
- Dessert: Baked Apples with Cinnamon

Day 7:

- Breakfast: Quinoa Breakfast Bowl
- Lunch: Chickpea and Spinach Curry
- Dinner: Cauliflower Pizza with Vegetables
- Snack: Mixed Berries Smoothie
- Dessert: Peanut Butter Banana Ice Cream

Week 2

Day 8:

- Breakfast: Veggie Breakfast Burrito
- Lunch: Greek Chicken Pita Wrap
- Dinner: Black Bean and Veggie Enchiladas
- Snack: Deviled Eggs with Avocado
- Dessert: Mixed Berry Crisp

Day 9:

- Breakfast: Smoothie Bowl with Greens
- Lunch: Zucchini Noodles with Pesto
- Dinner: Lemon Garlic Shrimp with Quinoa

- Snack: Baked Sweet Potato Fries
- Dessert: Chocolate Protein Balls

Day 10:

- Breakfast: Cottage Cheese and Fruit
- Lunch: Turkey and Avocado Wrap
- Dinner: Thai-Inspired Tofu Curry
- Snack: Caprese Skewers with Balsamic Glaze
- Dessert: Almond Butter Cookies

Day 11:

- Breakfast: Whole Grain Waffles with Nut Butter
- Lunch: Beef and Broccoli Stir-Fry
- Dinner: Eggplant Parmesan with Whole Wheat Pasta
- Snack: Spinach and Artichoke Dip (Lightened Up)
- Dessert: Mango and Coconut Rice Pudding

Day 12:

- Breakfast: Sweet Potato Hash with Turkey Sausage
- Lunch: Caprese Salad with Balsamic Glaze
- Dinner: Balsamic Glazed Chicken with Brussels Sprouts

- Snack: Quinoa and Black Bean Dip
- Dessert: Blueberry Protein Pancakes

Day 13:

- Breakfast: Overnight Oats with Peanut Butter
- Lunch: Sweet Potato and Chickpea Salad
- Dinner: Bison Chili with Kidney Beans
- Snack: Turkey and Avocado Roll-Ups
- Dessert: Chocolate-Dipped Strawberries

Day 14:

- Breakfast: Tofu Scramble with Veggies
- Lunch: Shrimp and Quinoa Bowl
- Dinner: Portobello Mushroom Steaks
- Snack: Sliced Apple with Almond Butter
- Dessert: Lemon Poppy Seed Cake

Week 3

Day 15:

- Breakfast: Pumpkin Pie Smoothie
- Lunch: Veggie and Hummus Wrap
- Dinner: Stuffed Zucchini Boats

- Snack: Greek Salad Skewers
- Dessert: Protein-Packed Cheesecake

Day 16:

- Breakfast: Protein Pancakes with Blueberries
- Lunch: Tofu and Vegetable Stir-Fry
- Dinner: Sesame Crusted Tuna Steak
- Snack: Smoked Salmon and Cucumber Bites
- Dessert: Oatmeal Raisin Energy Bites

Day 17:

- Breakfast: Breakfast Quiche with Spinach
- Lunch: Spinach and Feta Stuffed Chicken Breast
- Dinner: Beef and Broccoli Bowls
- Snack: Guacamole with Veggie Sticks
- Dessert: Raspberry Chia Jam

Day 18:

- Breakfast: High-Protein Breakfast Wrap
- Lunch: Rice Paper Spring Rolls with Peanut Sauce
- Dinner: Butternut Squash and Kale Risotto
- Snack: Hummus and Whole Wheat Pita

- Dessert: Chocolate Protein Balls

Day 19:

- Breakfast: Green Smoothie with Protein
- Lunch: Sweet Potato and Chickpea Salad
- Dinner: Spaghetti Squash with Turkey Meatballs
- Snack: Almonds and Dried Cranberries
- Dessert: Mixed Berry Crisp

Day 20:

- Breakfast: Chia Seed Pudding with Mango
- Lunch: Quinoa and Black Bean Bowl
- Dinner: Grilled Turkey Burgers with Sweet Potato Fries
- Snack: Greek Yogurt and Berries
- Dessert: Greek Yogurt Parfait with Honey

Day 21:

- Breakfast: Avocado Toast with Poached Egg
- Lunch: Salmon with Asparagus
- Dinner: Chicken and Vegetable Skewers
- Snack: Edamame with Sea Salt

- Dessert: Baked Apples with Cinnamon

Week 4

Day 22:

- Breakfast: Quinoa Breakfast Bowl
- Lunch: Chickpea and Spinach Curry
- Dinner: Cauliflower Pizza with Vegetables
- Snack: Mixed Berries Smoothie
- Dessert: Peanut Butter Banana Ice Cream

Day 23:

- Breakfast: Cottage Cheese and Fruit
- Lunch: Turkey and Avocado Wrap
- Dinner: Thai-Inspired Tofu Curry
- Snack: Caprese Skewers with Balsamic Glaze
- Dessert: Almond Butter Cookies

Day 24:

- Breakfast: Whole Grain Waffles with Nut Butter
- Lunch: Beef and Broccoli Stir-Fry
- Dinner: Eggplant Parmesan with Whole Wheat Pasta
- Snack: Spinach and Artichoke Dip (Lightened Up)

- Dessert: Mango and Coconut Rice Pudding

Day 25:

- Breakfast: Sweet Potato Hash with Turkey Sausage
- Lunch: Caprese Salad with Balsamic Glaze
- Dinner: Balsamic Glazed Chicken with Brussels Sprouts
- Snack: Quinoa and Black Bean Dip
- Dessert: Blueberry Protein Pancakes

Day 26:

- Breakfast: Overnight Oats with Peanut Butter
- Lunch: Sweet Potato and Chickpea Salad
- Dinner: Bison Chili with Kidney Beans
- Snack: Turkey and Avocado Roll-Ups
- Dessert: Chocolate-Dipped Strawberries

Day 27:

- Breakfast: Tofu Scramble with Veggies
- Lunch: Shrimp and Quinoa Bowl
- Dinner: Portobello Mushroom Steaks
- Snack: Sliced Apple with Almond Butter

- Dessert: Lemon Poppy Seed Cake

Day 28:

- Breakfast: Pumpkin Pie Smoothie
- Lunch: Veggie and Hummus Wrap
- Dinner: Stuffed Zucchini Boats
- Snack: Greek Salad Skewers
- Dessert: Protein-Packed Cheesecake

Day 29:

- Breakfast: High-Protein Breakfast Wrap
- Lunch: Rice Paper Spring Rolls with Peanut Sauce
- Dinner: Butternut Squash and Kale Risotto
- Snack: Hummus and Whole Wheat Pita
- Dessert: Chocolate Protein Balls

Day 30:

- Breakfast: Green Smoothie with Protein
- Lunch: Sweet Potato and Chickpea Salad
- Dinner: Spaghetti Squash with Turkey Meatballs
- Snack: Almonds and Dried Cranberries
- Dessert: Mixed Berry Crisp

Congratulations! You've completed a 30-day journey of healthy and delicious meals. Feel free to continue with this meal plan, repeat your favorite recipes, or modify it to suit your tastes and dietary requirements.

Chapter 2: Breakfast Recipes

Welcome to the delightful world of morning nourishment! In this chapter, we'll explore a diverse range of breakfast recipes that will kickstart your day with a burst of energy and flavor. From classic favorites to inventive creations, you'll find something to satisfy every palate.

Protein-Packed Scrambled Eggs

Ingredients:

- 2 large eggs
- 1/4 cup diced bell peppers
- 1/4 cup diced onions
- Salt and pepper to taste

Instructions:

1. Whisk eggs in a bowl.
2. Heat a non-stick skillet over medium heat and add diced vegetables.
3. Pour in whisked eggs and cook, stirring gently until scrambled. Season with salt and pepper.

Greek Yogurt Parfait with Berries

Ingredients:

- 1 cup Greek yogurt
- 1/2 cup mixed berries
- 1 tablespoon honey
- 2 tablespoons granola

Instructions:

1. In a glass, layer Greek yogurt, mixed berries, and honey.
2. Top with granola for added crunch.

Oatmeal with Almonds and Bananas

Ingredients:

- 1/2 cup rolled oats
- 1 cup almond milk
- 1/4 cup sliced almonds
- 1 ripe banana, sliced
- 1 teaspoon honey (optional)

Instructions:

1. Cook oats in almond milk until creamy.
2. Top with sliced almonds, banana, and a drizzle of honey if desired.

Spinach and Mushroom Omelette

Ingredients:

- 2 large eggs
- 1/2 cup chopped spinach
- 1/4 cup sliced mushrooms
- Salt and pepper to taste

Instructions:

1. Whisk eggs in a bowl.
2. Heat a skillet over medium heat, add spinach and mushrooms, and sauté until wilted.
3. Pour in whisked eggs, season, and cook until set.

Chia Seed Pudding with Mango

Ingredients:

- 2 tablespoons chia seeds

- 1/2 cup almond milk

- 1/2 cup diced mango

- 1 teaspoon maple syrup (optional)

Instructions:

1. Mix chia seeds and almond milk, let sit for 10 minutes.

2. Layer chia mixture with diced mango. Sweeten with maple syrup if desired.

Avocado Toast with Poached Egg

Ingredients:

- 1 slice whole grain bread

- 1/2 ripe avocado, mashed

- 1 poached egg

- Salt and pepper to taste

Instructions:

1. Toast the whole grain bread to your preference.

2. Spread mashed avocado on the toast.

3. Top with a perfectly poached egg, season with salt and pepper.

Quinoa Breakfast Bowl

Ingredients:

- 1/2 cup cooked quinoa
- 1/4 cup sliced strawberries
- 1/4 cup blueberries
- 2 tablespoons almond butter

Instructions:

1. Place cooked quinoa in a bowl.
2. Add sliced strawberries and blueberries.
3. Drizzle almond butter over the top for added flavor.

Protein Pancakes with Blueberries

Ingredients:

- 1/2 cup oats
- 1/2 cup cottage cheese
- 2 eggs
- 1/2 teaspoon baking powder
- 1/2 cup fresh blueberries

Instructions:

1. Blend oats, cottage cheese, eggs, and baking powder until smooth.

2. Pour onto a hot griddle and sprinkle with blueberries. Cook until bubbles form, then flip and cook the other side.

Veggie Breakfast Burrito

Ingredients:

- 1 whole wheat tortilla
- 2 eggs, scrambled
- 1/4 cup diced bell peppers
- 1/4 cup diced onions
- Salsa for garnish

Instructions:

1. Fill the tortilla with scrambled eggs, bell peppers, and onions.

2. Roll it up and serve with salsa on top.

Smoothie Bowl with Greens

Ingredients:

- 1 cup spinach or kale
- 1 frozen banana
- 1/2 cup almond milk
- Toppings: sliced banana, berries, granola, chia seeds

Instructions:

1. Blend spinach or kale, frozen banana, and almond milk until smooth.
2. Pour into a bowl and add your favorite toppings.

Cottage Cheese and Fruit

Ingredients:

- 1 cup low-fat cottage cheese
- 1/2 cup mixed fresh fruit (e.g., strawberries, kiwi, and pineapple)
- 1 tablespoon honey (optional)

Instructions:

1. Spoon cottage cheese into a bowl.

2. Top with mixed fresh fruit and drizzle with honey for sweetness.

Whole Grain Waffles with Nut Butter

Ingredients:

- 2 whole grain waffles
- 2 tablespoons almond or peanut butter
- Sliced banana for topping

Instructions:

1. Toast the whole grain waffles.
2. Spread almond or peanut butter on top.
3. Add sliced banana for extra flavor.

Sweet Potato Hash with Turkey Sausage

Ingredients:

- 1 sweet potato, diced
- 1/4 cup diced turkey sausage
- 1/4 cup diced bell peppers
- Salt and pepper to taste

Instructions:

1. Heat a skillet over medium heat.

2. Add sweet potato, turkey sausage, and bell peppers.
    Cook until sweet potatoes are tender and sausage is
    browned.

Overnight Oats with Peanut Butter

Ingredients:

- 1/2 cup rolled oats
- 1/2 cup almond milk
- 1 tablespoon peanut butter
- 1/2 banana, sliced

Instructions:

1. Mix rolled oats and almond milk in a jar. Refrigerate
    overnight.

2. In the morning, top with peanut butter and banana
    slices.

Tofu Scramble with Veggies

Ingredients:

- 1/2 cup crumbled tofu
- 1/4 cup diced tomatoes
- 1/4 cup diced bell peppers
- 1/4 cup diced onions
- Turmeric, cumin, and salt to taste

Instructions:

1. In a skillet, sauté tofu, tomatoes, bell peppers, and onions.
2. Season with turmeric, cumin, and salt to taste.

Breakfast Quiche with Spinach

Ingredients:

- 4 large eggs
- 1 cup chopped spinach
- 1/4 cup diced tomatoes
- 1/4 cup shredded cheddar cheese

Instructions:

1. Whisk eggs in a bowl.
2. In a greased baking dish, layer spinach, tomatoes, and cheese. Pour eggs over the top.
3. Bake until set and lightly browned.

High-Protein Breakfast Wrap

Ingredients:

- 1 whole wheat tortilla
- 2 scrambled eggs
- 1/4 cup black beans
- Salsa and sliced avocado for garnish

Instructions:

1. Fill the tortilla with scrambled eggs and black beans.
2. Top with salsa and sliced avocado.

Green Smoothie with Protein

Ingredients:

- 1 cup spinach
- 1/2 cup Greek yogurt

- 1/2 banana

- 1 scoop of your favorite protein powder

- 1/2 cup almond milk

Instructions:

1. Blend spinach, Greek yogurt, banana, protein powder, and almond milk until smooth.

Chapter 3: Lunch Recipes

In this chapter, we explore a delightful array of lunch recipes that not only tantalize your taste buds but also keep you on track with your healthy macro diet. These recipes are designed to provide you with a balanced mix of protein, carbohydrates, and healthy fats, ensuring you stay satisfied and energized throughout the day.

Grilled Chicken Salad with Avocado

Ingredients:

- 2 boneless, skinless chicken breasts
- 1 avocado, sliced
- Mixed greens
- Cherry tomatoes, halved
- Red onion, thinly sliced
- Olive oil
- Lemon juice
- Salt and pepper to taste

Instructions:

1. Preheat the grill to medium-high heat.
2. Season chicken breasts with salt, pepper, and a drizzle of olive oil.
3. Grill chicken for about 6-7 minutes per side until cooked through.
4. Slice chicken into strips.
5. In a large bowl, combine mixed greens, cherry tomatoes, red onion, and avocado.
6. Drizzle with olive oil and lemon juice.
7. Top with grilled chicken strips.
8. Season with salt and pepper to taste.

Quinoa and Black Bean Bowl

Ingredients:

- 1 cup cooked quinoa
- 1 can black beans, drained and rinsed
- Corn kernels
- Red bell pepper, diced
- Red onion, finely chopped
- Cilantro, chopped
- Lime juice

- Olive oil
- Salt and pepper to taste

Instructions:

1. In a large bowl, combine cooked quinoa, black beans, corn, red bell pepper, and red onion.
2. In a separate bowl, whisk together lime juice, olive oil, cilantro, salt, and pepper.
3. Pour the dressing over the quinoa mixture and toss to combine.

Tuna Salad Lettuce Wraps

Ingredients:

- Canned tuna in water, drained
- Greek yogurt
- Dijon mustard
- Celery, finely chopped
- Red onion, finely chopped
- Lettuce leaves for wrapping

Instructions:

1. In a bowl, mix canned tuna, Greek yogurt, Dijon mustard, celery, and red onion.

2. Spoon the tuna salad mixture onto lettuce leaves.

3. Wrap and enjoy!

Turkey and Veggie Stir-Fry

Ingredients:

- Ground turkey
- Mixed vegetables (bell peppers, broccoli, carrots)
- Low-sodium soy sauce
- Garlic, minced
- Ginger, minced
- Olive oil

Instructions:

1. Heat olive oil in a pan and cook ground turkey until browned.

2. Add minced garlic and ginger, stir for a minute.

3. Add mixed vegetables and soy sauce.

4. Stir-fry until vegetables are tender and the turkey is cooked through.

Lentil Soup with Spinach

Ingredients:

- Green or brown lentils
- Vegetable broth
- Spinach leaves
- Carrots, diced
- Celery, diced
- Onion, diced
- Garlic, minced
- Olive oil
- Spices (cumin, paprika, salt, and pepper)

Instructions:

1. Heat olive oil in a pot and sauté onions, garlic, carrots, and celery until softened.
2. Add lentils, vegetable broth, and spices.
3. Simmer until lentils are tender.
4. Stir in spinach leaves until wilted.

Salmon with Asparagus

Ingredients:

- Salmon fillets
- Asparagus spears
- Lemon slices
- Olive oil
- Garlic powder
- Salt and pepper

Instructions:

1. Preheat the oven to 375°F (190°C).
2. Place salmon fillets and asparagus on a baking sheet.
3. Drizzle with olive oil and sprinkle with garlic powder, salt, and pepper.
4. Top with lemon slices.
5. Bake for 15-20 minutes until salmon flakes easily.

Chickpea and Spinach Curry

Ingredients:

- Chickpeas
- Spinach leaves

- Coconut milk

- Curry paste

- Onion, diced

- Garlic, minced

- Olive oil

- Spices (coriander, cumin, turmeric, salt)

Instructions:

1. Heat olive oil in a pan, sauté onions and garlic until fragrant.
2. Add curry paste and spices, cook for a minute.
3. Stir in chickpeas, spinach, and coconut milk.
4. Simmer until spinach wilts and flavors meld.

Greek Chicken Pita Wrap

Ingredients:

- Grilled chicken breast, sliced

- Whole wheat pita bread

- Greek yogurt tzatziki sauce

- Cherry tomatoes, halved

- Cucumber, sliced

- Red onion, thinly sliced

- Fresh mint leaves

Instructions:

1. Warm pita bread.
2. Spread tzatziki sauce on the pita.
3. Add sliced chicken, cherry tomatoes, cucumber, red onion, and mint leaves.
4. Roll it up and enjoy!

Zucchini Noodles with Pesto

Ingredients:

- Zucchini, spiralized into noodles
- Basil pesto sauce (store-bought or homemade)
- Cherry tomatoes, halved
- Parmesan cheese (optional)
- Pine nuts (optional)

Instructions:

1. Spiralize zucchini into noodles.
2. Toss zucchini noodles with basil pesto sauce.
3. Add cherry tomatoes and, if desired, sprinkle with Parmesan cheese and pine nuts.

Turkey and Avocado Wrap

Ingredients:

- Whole wheat tortilla wraps
- Sliced turkey breast
- Avocado slices
- Lettuce leaves
- Tomato slices
- Dijon mustard (optional)

Instructions:

1. Lay out a tortilla wrap.
2. Layer sliced turkey, avocado, lettuce, tomato, and a drizzle of Dijon mustard (if desired).
3. Roll up the wrap and enjoy!

Beef and Broccoli Stir-Fry

Ingredients:

- Lean beef strips
- Broccoli florets
- Low-sodium soy sauce
- Garlic, minced

- Ginger, minced
- Olive oil
- Brown rice (optional)

Instructions:

1. Heat olive oil in a pan and stir-fry beef until browned.
2. Add minced garlic and ginger, stir for a minute.
3. Add broccoli and soy sauce.
4. Stir-fry until broccoli is tender.
5. Serve over brown rice if desired.

Caprese Salad with Balsamic Glaze

Ingredients:

- Fresh mozzarella cheese, sliced
- Tomatoes, sliced
- Fresh basil leaves
- Balsamic glaze
- Olive oil
- Salt and pepper

Instructions:

1. Arrange mozzarella, tomato, and basil slices on a
    plate.
2. Drizzle with olive oil and balsamic glaze.
3. Season with salt and pepper.

Sweet Potato and Chickpea Salad

Ingredients:

- Roasted sweet potatoes
- Chickpeas
- Red onion, finely chopped
- Cilantro, chopped
- Olive oil
- Lemon juice
- Salt and pepper

Instructions:

1. Combine roasted sweet potatoes, chickpeas, red
    onion, and cilantro in a bowl.
2. Drizzle with olive oil and lemon juice.
3. Season with salt and pepper.

Shrimp and Quinoa Bowl

Ingredients:

- Cooked shrimp
- Cooked quinoa
- Avocado slices
- Cherry tomatoes, halved
- Cucumber, diced
- Fresh cilantro leaves
- Lime juice
- Olive oil
- Salt and pepper

Instructions:

1. In a bowl, combine cooked shrimp, quinoa, avocado, cherry tomatoes, cucumber, and cilantro.
2. Drizzle with olive oil and lime juice.
3. Season with salt and pepper to taste.

Veggie and Hummus Wrap

Ingredients:

- Whole wheat tortilla wraps

- Hummus
- Sliced bell peppers
- Sliced cucumber
- Sliced carrots
- Spinach leaves

Instructions:

1. Spread a layer of hummus on a whole wheat tortilla.
2. Add sliced bell peppers, cucumber, carrots, and spinach leaves.
3. Roll up the wrap and enjoy!

Tofu and Vegetable Stir-Fry

Ingredients:

- Extra-firm tofu, cubed
- Mixed vegetables (broccoli, bell peppers, snap peas)
- Low-sodium stir-fry sauce
- Garlic, minced
- Ginger, minced
- Olive oil
- Brown rice (optional)

Instructions:

1. Heat olive oil in a pan and stir-fry tofu until golden.

2. Add minced garlic and ginger, stir for a minute.

3. Add mixed vegetables and stir-fry sauce.

4. Stir-fry until vegetables are tender.

5. Serve over brown rice if desired.

Spinach and Feta Stuffed Chicken Breast

Ingredients:

- Boneless, skinless chicken breasts
- Fresh spinach leaves
- Feta cheese crumbles
- Olive oil
- Garlic powder
- Salt and pepper

Instructions:

1. Preheat the oven to 375°F (190°C).

2. Butterfly chicken breasts and stuff with spinach and feta.

3. Drizzle with olive oil and season with garlic powder, salt, and pepper.

4. Bake for 25-30 minutes until chicken is cooked through.

Rice Paper Spring Rolls with Peanut Sauce

Ingredients:

- Rice paper wrappers
- Cooked shrimp or tofu strips
- Rice vermicelli noodles
- Cucumber, carrot, and bell pepper strips
- Fresh mint leaves
- Peanut sauce for dipping

Instructions:

1. Dip a rice paper wrapper in warm water to soften.

2. Lay it flat and add shrimp or tofu, rice noodles, veggies, and mint leaves.

3. Roll up the wrapper, tucking in the sides as you go.

4. Serve with peanut sauce for dipping.

Chapter 4: Dinner Recipes

Welcome to the heart of your journey towards healthy eating. In this chapter, we present an array of delightful dinner recipes that are not only delicious but also packed with the nutrients your body craves. Each dish is carefully crafted to support your macro diet goals while tantalizing your taste buds.

Baked Salmon with Lemon and Dill

Ingredients:

- 4 salmon fillets
- 2 tablespoons olive oil
- 2 lemons, thinly sliced
- 2 tablespoons fresh dill
- Salt and pepper to taste

Instructions:

1. Preheat your oven to 375°F (190°C).
2. Place salmon fillets on a baking sheet.

3. Drizzle olive oil over the salmon and season with salt and pepper.

4. Arrange lemon slices on top of the fillets and sprinkle with fresh dill.

5. Bake for 15-20 minutes until the salmon flakes easily with a fork.

Grilled Turkey Burgers with Sweet Potato Fries

Ingredients:

- 1 lb ground turkey
- 1/4 cup diced onions
- 1/4 cup diced bell peppers
- 1/2 teaspoon garlic powder
- Salt and pepper to taste
- Sweet potato fries (store-bought or homemade)

Instructions:

1. In a bowl, combine ground turkey, onions, bell peppers, garlic powder, salt, and pepper.

2. Shape the mixture into burger patties.

3. Grill the turkey burgers until cooked through (about 4-5 minutes per side).

4. Serve with sweet potato fries.

Quinoa-Stuffed Bell Peppers

Ingredients:

- 4 bell peppers, any color
- 1 cup quinoa, rinsed
- 2 cups vegetable broth
- 1 cup diced tomatoes
- 1 cup black beans, drained and rinsed
- 1/2 cup corn kernels
- 1 teaspoon chili powder
- 1/2 teaspoon cumin
- Salt and pepper to taste

Instructions:

1. Cut the tops off the bell peppers and remove the seeds.

2. In a saucepan, combine quinoa and vegetable broth. Bring to a boil, then reduce heat and simmer for 15 minutes.

3. In a bowl, mix cooked quinoa, diced tomatoes, black beans, corn, chili powder, cumin, salt, and pepper.

4. Stuff each bell pepper with the quinoa mixture.

5. Bake at 350°F (175°C) for 25-30 minutes until peppers are tender.

Spaghetti Squash with Turkey Meatballs

Ingredients:

- 1 spaghetti squash, halved and seeded
- 1 lb ground turkey
- 1/4 cup breadcrumbs
- 1/4 cup grated Parmesan cheese
- 1 egg
- 1 cup marinara sauce
- Fresh basil leaves for garnish
- Salt and pepper to taste

Instructions:

1. Preheat your oven to 375°F (190°C).

2. Place spaghetti squash halves on a baking sheet, cut side down. Bake for 30-40 minutes until tender.

3. In a bowl, combine ground turkey, breadcrumbs, Parmesan cheese, egg, salt, and pepper. Form into meatballs.

4. Heat marinara sauce in a large skillet, then add meatballs and simmer until cooked through.

5. Scrape the cooked spaghetti squash with a fork to create "noodles."

6. Serve meatballs and sauce over spaghetti squash. Garnish with fresh basil.

Teriyaki Tofu Stir-Fry

Ingredients:

- 1 block of extra-firm tofu, cubed
- 2 tablespoons teriyaki sauce
- 1 tablespoon sesame oil
- 2 cups broccoli florets
- 1 red bell pepper, sliced
- 1 cup snap peas
- 2 cloves garlic, minced
- Cooked brown rice for serving

Instructions:

1. In a bowl, marinate the cubed tofu in teriyaki sauce for about 10 minutes.
2. Heat sesame oil in a large skillet over medium-high heat.
3. Add marinated tofu and cook until golden brown.
4. Add broccoli, red bell pepper, snap peas, and minced garlic to the skillet. Stir-fry until vegetables are tender.
5. Serve over cooked brown rice.

Chicken and Vegetable Skewers

Ingredients:

- 1 lb chicken breast, cut into chunks
- 1 zucchini, sliced
- 1 red onion, sliced
- 1 red bell pepper, cut into squares
- 1/4 cup olive oil
- 2 tablespoons lemon juice
- 1 teaspoon dried oregano
- Salt and pepper to taste

Instructions:

1. In a bowl, combine olive oil, lemon juice, dried oregano, salt, and pepper.
2. Thread chicken and vegetables onto skewers.
3. Brush skewers with the olive oil mixture.
4. Grill or broil the skewers until the chicken is cooked through and vegetables are tender.

Cauliflower Pizza with Vegetables

Ingredients:

- 1 cauliflower pizza crust (store-bought or homemade)
- 1/2 cup pizza sauce
- 1 cup shredded mozzarella cheese
- Assorted vegetable toppings (e.g., bell peppers, mushrooms, spinach)
- Fresh basil leaves for garnish

Instructions:

1. Preheat your oven according to the cauliflower crust instructions.
2. Spread pizza sauce over the cauliflower crust.

3. Sprinkle with mozzarella cheese and add your favorite vegetable toppings.

4. Bake until the crust is golden and the cheese is melted and bubbly.

5. Garnish with fresh basil leaves before serving.

Black Bean and Veggie Enchiladas

Ingredients:

- 8 whole wheat tortillas
- 2 cups cooked black beans
- 1 cup diced bell peppers
- 1 cup corn kernels
- 1 cup diced tomatoes
- 1 cup diced onions
- 1 teaspoon chili powder
- 1/2 teaspoon cumin
- 1 cup enchilada sauce
- 1 cup shredded cheddar cheese

Instructions:

1. Preheat your oven to 350°F (175°C).

2. In a large skillet, sauté onions, bell peppers, corn, and tomatoes until tender. Add black beans, chili powder, and cumin.

3. Spoon the black bean mixture onto each tortilla, roll them up, and place them in a baking dish.

4. Pour enchilada sauce over the rolled tortillas and top with shredded cheddar cheese.

5. Bake for 20-25 minutes until the cheese is bubbly and enchiladas are heated through.

Lemon Garlic Shrimp with Quinoa

Ingredients:

- 1 lb large shrimp, peeled and deveined
- 2 cups cooked quinoa
- 2 tablespoons olive oil
- 3 cloves garlic, minced
- Zest and juice of 1 lemon
- 1/4 cup fresh parsley, chopped
- Salt and pepper to taste

Instructions:

1. Heat olive oil in a skillet over medium-high heat.

2. Add minced garlic and cook for about 1 minute until fragrant.

3. Add shrimp and cook until they turn pink and opaque, about 2-3 minutes per side.

4. Stir in lemon zest, lemon juice, and chopped parsley.

5. Serve over cooked quinoa.

Thai-Inspired Tofu Curry

Ingredients:

- 1 block of tofu, cubed
- 1 can coconut milk
- 2 tablespoons red curry paste
- 2 cups mixed vegetables (e.g., bell peppers, broccoli, carrots)
- 1 tablespoon soy sauce
- 1 tablespoon brown sugar
- Cooked jasmine rice for serving

Instructions:

1. In a large skillet, heat coconut milk and red curry paste over medium heat.

2. Add cubed tofu and mixed vegetables. Simmer until vegetables are tender.

3. Stir in soy sauce and brown sugar.

4. Serve over cooked jasmine rice.

Eggplant Parmesan with Whole Wheat Pasta

Ingredients:

- 2 large eggplants, sliced
- 2 cups whole wheat pasta
- 2 cups marinara sauce
- 1 cup shredded mozzarella cheese
- 1/4 cup grated Parmesan cheese
- Fresh basil leaves for garnish
- Olive oil for frying

Instructions:

1. Heat olive oil in a large skillet over medium-high heat.

2. Fry eggplant slices until golden brown, then drain on paper towels.

3. Cook whole wheat pasta according to package instructions.

4. In a baking dish, layer cooked pasta, marinara sauce, fried eggplant slices, mozzarella cheese, and Parmesan cheese.

5. Bake at 375°F (190°C) for 20-25 minutes until bubbly and cheese is melted.

6. Garnish with fresh basil before serving.

Balsamic Glazed Chicken with Brussels Sprouts

Ingredients:

- 4 boneless, skinless chicken breasts
- 2 cups Brussels sprouts, halved
- 1/4 cup balsamic vinegar
- 2 tablespoons honey
- 2 cloves garlic, minced
- Salt and pepper to taste

Instructions:

1. Season chicken breasts with salt and pepper.

2. In a skillet, sear chicken until golden brown and cooked through.

3. In the same skillet, add halved Brussels sprouts and minced garlic. Sauté until tender.

4. In a small bowl, mix balsamic vinegar and honey. Drizzle over chicken and Brussels sprouts.

5. Serve hot.

Bison Chili with Kidney Beans

Ingredients:

- 1 lb ground bison
- 1 onion, diced
- 2 cloves garlic, minced
- 1 can kidney beans, drained and rinsed
- 1 can diced tomatoes
- 2 tablespoons chili powder
- 1 teaspoon cumin
- Salt and pepper to taste

Instructions:

1. In a large pot, brown ground bison over medium-high heat.

2. Add diced onions and minced garlic. Cook until onions are translucent.

3. Stir in kidney beans, diced tomatoes, chili powder, cumin, salt, and pepper.

4. Simmer for about 20 minutes until flavors meld together.

Portobello Mushroom Steaks

Ingredients:

- 4 large Portobello mushrooms
- 2 tablespoons olive oil
- 2 cloves garlic, minced
- 2 tablespoons balsamic vinegar
- Fresh thyme leaves for garnish
- Salt and pepper to taste

Instructions:

1. Preheat your grill or oven to medium-high heat.
2. Clean Portobello mushrooms and remove stems.
3. In a bowl, mix olive oil, minced garlic, balsamic vinegar, salt, and pepper.
4. Brush the mushroom caps with the olive oil mixture.

5. Grill or bake for about 10 minutes per side until tender.

6. Garnish with fresh thyme leaves.

Stuffed Zucchini Boats

Ingredients:

- 4 zucchini
- 1 lb ground turkey
- 1/2 cup diced onions
- 1/2 cup diced bell peppers
- 1/2 cup diced tomatoes
- 1/2 cup shredded mozzarella cheese
- 1/2 teaspoon Italian seasoning
- Salt and pepper to taste

Instructions:

1. Preheat your oven to 375°F (190°C).

2. Cut zucchini in half lengthwise and scoop out the centers to create "boats."

3. In a skillet, cook ground turkey, onions, bell peppers, and diced tomatoes until turkey is browned.

4. Stir in Italian seasoning, salt, and pepper.

5. Fill the zucchini boats with the turkey mixture.

6. Sprinkle with shredded mozzarella cheese.

7. Bake for 20-25 minutes until zucchini is tender and cheese is melted.

Sesame Crusted Tuna Steak

Ingredients:

- 4 tuna steaks
- 1/4 cup sesame seeds
- 1/4 cup soy sauce
- 2 tablespoons honey
- 2 cloves garlic, minced
- 1 tablespoon sesame oil
- Salt and pepper to taste

Instructions:

1. In a shallow dish, spread sesame seeds.

2. Coat tuna steaks in sesame seeds, pressing to adhere.

3. In a bowl, mix soy sauce, honey, minced garlic, sesame oil, salt, and pepper.

4. Grill or sear tuna steaks for about 2-3 minutes per side for medium-rare.

5. Drizzle with the soy sauce mixture before serving.

Beef and Broccoli Bowls

Ingredients:

- 1 lb beef sirloin, thinly sliced
- 2 cups broccoli florets
- 1/4 cup soy sauce
- 2 tablespoons brown sugar
- 2 cloves garlic, minced
- Cooked brown rice for serving

Instructions:

1. In a bowl, mix soy sauce, brown sugar, and minced garlic.
2. In a skillet, sear beef slices until browned. Remove from skillet.
3. Add broccoli florets to the skillet and stir-fry until tender.
4. Return beef to the skillet and pour the soy sauce mixture over it.
5. Serve over cooked brown rice.

Butternut Squash and Kale Risotto

Ingredients:

- 2 cups arborio rice
- 4 cups vegetable broth
- 1 butternut squash, diced
- 2 cups kale, chopped
- 1/2 cup grated Parmesan cheese
- 2 tablespoons olive oil
- Salt and pepper to taste

Instructions:

1. In a large pot, heat olive oil over medium heat.
2. Add arborio rice and stir until lightly toasted.
3. Gradually add vegetable broth, one cup at a time, stirring until absorbed.
4. Stir in diced butternut squash and continue to cook until rice is tender.
5. Add chopped kale and cook until wilted.
6. Stir in grated Parmesan cheese, salt, and pepper.

Chapter 5: Snacks and Appetizers

In Chapter 5 of your "Healthy Macro Diet Meal Plans," we're diving into the world of delicious and nutritious snacks and appetizers. These recipes are designed to keep your energy up and your cravings satisfied throughout the day. Below, you'll find a collection of delectable options that are perfect for any occasion.

Guacamole with Veggie Sticks

Ingredients:

- 2 ripe avocados
- 1 small onion, finely diced
- 2 cloves garlic, minced
- 1 tomato, diced
- 1 lime, juiced
- Salt and pepper to taste
- Assorted veggie sticks (carrots, cucumbers, bell peppers)

Instructions:

1. Cut the avocados in half, remove the pit, and scoop the flesh into a bowl.
2. Mash the avocados with a fork until you achieve your desired guacamole consistency.
3. Add the diced onion, minced garlic, diced tomato, and lime juice to the mashed avocado. Mix well.
4. Season with salt and pepper to taste.
5. Serve with a colorful assortment of veggie sticks for dipping.

Hummus and Whole Wheat Pita

Ingredients:

- Whole wheat pita bread
- Store-bought or homemade hummus

Instructions:

1. Cut the whole wheat pita into triangles or strips.
2. Serve with a generous portion of your favorite hummus for dipping.

Almonds and Dried Cranberries

Ingredients:

- Almonds
- Dried cranberries

Instructions:

1. Mix a handful of almonds with an equal amount of dried cranberries.
2. Portion into small snack-sized bags for easy, on-the-go munching.

Greek Yogurt and Berries

Ingredients:

- Greek yogurt
- Fresh berries (strawberries, blueberries, raspberries)

Instructions:

1. Spoon Greek yogurt into a bowl.
2. Top with a handful of fresh berries for a burst of flavor and antioxidants.

Cottage Cheese with Pineapple

Ingredients:

- Cottage cheese
- Fresh or canned pineapple chunks

Instructions:

1. Spoon cottage cheese into a bowl.
2. Add pineapple chunks on top for a sweet and savory snack.

Trail Mix with Nuts and Seeds

Ingredients:

- Almonds
- Walnuts
- Pumpkin seeds
- Sunflower seeds
- Raisins
- Dried apricots

Instructions:

1. Combine a mix of almonds, walnuts, pumpkin seeds, sunflower seeds, raisins, and chopped dried apricots in a bowl.
2. Toss everything together and portion into snack-sized containers for a crunchy and energy-boosting treat.

Sliced Cucumber with Tzatziki

Ingredients:

- Cucumber, thinly sliced
- Tzatziki sauce (store-bought or homemade)

Instructions:

1. Slice the cucumber into thin rounds.
2. Dip the cucumber slices into tzatziki sauce for a refreshing and tangy snack.

Edamame with Sea Salt

Ingredients:

- Edamame (frozen or fresh)

- Sea salt

Instructions:

1. Cook the edamame according to package instructions.
2. Sprinkle with sea salt and enjoy these protein-packed little green gems.

Mixed Berries Smoothie

Ingredients:

- Mixed berries (strawberries, blueberries, raspberries)
- Greek yogurt
- Honey (optional)

Instructions:

1. Blend mixed berries with Greek yogurt until smooth.
2. Add a drizzle of honey if desired for extra sweetness.

Deviled Eggs with Avocado

Ingredients:

- Hard-boiled eggs, cut in half

- Avocado, mashed
- Dijon mustard
- Paprika
- Chopped chives

Instructions:

1. Remove yolks from the hard-boiled eggs and mix them with mashed avocado and a touch of Dijon mustard.
2. Fill the egg whites with the avocado mixture.
3. Sprinkle with paprika and garnish with chopped chives.

Baked Sweet Potato Fries

Ingredients:

- Sweet potatoes, cut into fries
- Olive oil
- Paprika
- Salt and pepper

Instructions:

1. Preheat your oven to 425°F (220°C).

2. Toss sweet potato fries with olive oil, paprika, salt, and pepper.

3. Spread them out on a baking sheet in a single layer.

4. Bake for about 25-30 minutes until they are crispy and golden brown.

Caprese Skewers with Balsamic Glaze

Ingredients:

- Cherry tomatoes
- Fresh mozzarella balls
- Fresh basil leaves
- Balsamic glaze

Instructions:

1. Assemble cherry tomatoes, mozzarella balls, and fresh basil leaves on skewers.

2. Drizzle with balsamic glaze for a flavorful bite-sized treat.

Spinach and Artichoke Dip (Lightened Up)

Ingredients:

- Spinach, cooked and chopped
- Artichoke hearts, chopped
- Greek yogurt
- Parmesan cheese
- Garlic powder
- Salt and pepper

Instructions:

1. Mix cooked and chopped spinach and artichoke hearts with Greek yogurt, Parmesan cheese, garlic powder, salt, and pepper.
2. Serve as a dip with veggie sticks or whole wheat crackers.

Quinoa and Black Bean Dip

Ingredients:

- Cooked quinoa
- Black beans, drained and rinsed

- Salsa

- Lime juice

- Cilantro, chopped

Instructions:

1. Combine cooked quinoa, black beans, salsa, lime juice, and chopped cilantro.

2. Serve as a dip or a side dish with whole wheat pita or tortilla chips.

Turkey and Avocado Roll-Ups

Ingredients:

- Sliced turkey breast

- Avocado slices

- Baby spinach leaves

- Mustard (optional)

Instructions:

1. Lay out a slice of turkey breast and top with avocado slices and baby spinach leaves.

2. Add a touch of mustard if desired, then roll up for a quick and satisfying snack.

Sliced Apple with Almond Butter

Ingredients:

- Apple, thinly sliced
- Almond butter

Instructions:

1. Slice the apple into thin pieces.
2. Pair the apple slices with almond butter for a satisfying combination of crunch and creaminess.

Greek Salad Skewers

Ingredients:

- Cherry tomatoes
- Cucumber, diced
- Feta cheese, cubed
- Kalamata olives
- Red onion, finely chopped
- Greek salad dressing

Instructions:

1. Thread cherry tomatoes, cucumber, feta cheese, Kalamata olives, and red onion onto skewers.

2. Drizzle with Greek salad dressing for a taste of the Mediterranean.

Smoked Salmon and Cucumber Bites

Ingredients:

- Cucumber slices
- Smoked salmon
- Cream cheese
- Fresh dill

Instructions:

1. Spread a small amount of cream cheese on each cucumber slice.

2. Top with a piece of smoked salmon and garnish with fresh dill for an elegant and tasty appetizer.

Chapter 6: Desserts

In this chapter, we present you with a collection of delectable desserts that not only satisfy your sweet tooth but also align with your macro diet goals. From rich and chocolaty creations to fruity delights and protein-packed treats, these recipes will leave you craving more while keeping your macros in check.

Dark Chocolate Avocado Mousse

Ingredients:

- 2 ripe avocados
- 1/4 cup dark cocoa powder
- 1/4 cup honey or maple syrup
- 1 tsp vanilla extract
- A pinch of salt

Instructions:

1. Blend avocados, cocoa powder, honey or maple syrup, vanilla extract, and a pinch of salt until smooth.

2. Chill for at least 30 minutes before serving.

Greek Yogurt Parfait with Honey

Ingredients:

- 1 cup Greek yogurt
- 1/2 cup fresh mixed berries
- 2 tbsp honey
- 2 tbsp granola (optional)

Instructions:

1. Layer Greek yogurt, mixed berries, honey, and granola (if desired) in a glass or bowl.
2. Enjoy this simple and satisfying parfait.

Berry Sorbet

Ingredients:

- 2 cups frozen mixed berries
- 1/4 cup honey
- 1 tbsp lemon juice

Instructions:

1. Blend frozen berries, honey, and lemon juice until smooth.

2. Freeze for a couple of hours, then scoop and serve.

Protein-Packed Chocolate Brownies

Ingredients:

- 1 cup black beans (canned, drained, and rinsed)
- 1/2 cup chocolate protein powder
- 1/4 cup cocoa powder
- 1/4 cup honey
- 1/4 cup almond butter
- 1 tsp vanilla extract

Instructions:

1. Blend black beans, protein powder, cocoa powder, honey, almond butter, and vanilla extract until well combined.

2. Bake in a greased pan at 350°F (175°C) for 20-25 minutes.

Chia Seed Pudding with Cocoa

Ingredients:

- 3 tbsp chia seeds
- 1 cup almond milk
- 2 tbsp cocoa powder
- 2 tbsp honey or maple syrup
- 1/2 tsp vanilla extract

Instructions:

1. Mix chia seeds, almond milk, cocoa powder, honey or maple syrup, and vanilla extract in a jar.
2. Refrigerate overnight, stirring occasionally, until it reaches a pudding-like consistency.

Baked Apples with Cinnamon

Ingredients:

- 4 apples, cored and halved
- 1 tsp cinnamon
- 2 tbsp honey or maple syrup
- 1/4 cup chopped walnuts (optional)

Instructions:

1. Preheat your oven to 350°F (175°C).

2. Place apple halves in a baking dish, sprinkle with cinnamon, drizzle with honey or maple syrup, and add chopped walnuts if desired.

3. Bake for about 25-30 minutes until apples are tender and caramelized.

Peanut Butter Banana Ice Cream

Ingredients:

- 4 ripe bananas, frozen
- 2 tbsp peanut butter
- 1 tsp vanilla extract

Instructions:

1. Blend frozen bananas, peanut butter, and vanilla extract until creamy.

2. Freeze for an hour for a firmer texture.

Mixed Berry Crisp

Ingredients:

- 2 cups mixed berries (strawberries, blueberries, raspberries)
- 1/2 cup oats
- 1/4 cup almond flour
- 2 tbsp honey or maple syrup
- 1 tsp cinnamon

Instructions:

1. Combine mixed berries in a baking dish.
2. In a separate bowl, mix oats, almond flour, honey or maple syrup, and cinnamon. Sprinkle this mixture over the berries.
3. Bake at 350°F (175°C) for 20-25 minutes until the top is golden brown.

Chocolate Protein Balls

Ingredients:

- 1 cup rolled oats
- 1/2 cup chocolate protein powder

- 1/2 cup almond butter
- 1/4 cup honey
- 1/4 cup dark chocolate chips

Instructions:

1. Mix rolled oats, protein powder, almond butter, honey, and dark chocolate chips in a bowl.
2. Roll the mixture into bite-sized balls and refrigerate for 30 minutes.

Almond Butter Cookies

Ingredients:

- 1 cup almond butter
- 1/4 cup honey
- 1 egg
- 1/2 tsp baking soda
- 1/2 tsp vanilla extract

Instructions:

1. Preheat your oven to 350°F (175°C).
2. Mix almond butter, honey, egg, baking soda, and vanilla extract in a bowl.

3. Drop spoonfuls of dough onto a baking sheet and bake for 10-12 minutes.

Mango and Coconut Rice Pudding

Ingredients:

- 1 cup cooked brown rice
- 1 cup coconut milk
- 1 ripe mango, diced
- 2 tbsp honey or maple syrup
- 1/2 tsp vanilla extract

Instructions:

1. In a saucepan, combine cooked brown rice, coconut milk, honey or maple syrup, and vanilla extract.
2. Simmer over low heat, stirring occasionally, until the mixture thickens.
3. Top with diced mango before serving.

Blueberry Protein Pancakes

Ingredients:

- 1 cup rolled oats

- 1 scoop blueberry protein powder
- 1/2 cup Greek yogurt
- 2 eggs
- 1/2 tsp baking powder
- 1/2 cup fresh blueberries

Instructions:

1. Blend rolled oats, blueberry protein powder, Greek yogurt, eggs, and baking powder until smooth.
2. Fold in fresh blueberries.
3. Cook pancakes on a griddle over medium heat until golden brown on both sides.

Chocolate-Dipped Strawberries

Ingredients:

- 12 fresh strawberries
- 1/4 cup dark chocolate chips
- 1 tsp coconut oil

Instructions:

1. Melt dark chocolate chips and coconut oil in a microwave-safe bowl.

2. Dip strawberries into the melted chocolate and place them on a parchment-lined tray.

3. Allow the chocolate to set in the refrigerator.

Lemon Poppy Seed Cake

Ingredients:

- 1 1/2 cups almond flour
- 1/4 cup coconut flour
- 1/4 cup honey or maple syrup
- 1/4 cup lemon juice
- Zest of one lemon
- 3 eggs
- 2 tbsp poppy seeds
- 1/2 tsp baking soda

Instructions:

1. Preheat your oven to 350°F (175°C).

2. Mix almond flour, coconut flour, honey or maple syrup, lemon juice, lemon zest, eggs, poppy seeds, and baking soda.

3. Pour the batter into a greased baking pan and bake for 25-30 minutes.

Pumpkin Pie Smoothie

Ingredients:

- 1 cup pumpkin puree
- 1/2 cup Greek yogurt
- 1/2 cup almond milk
- 1 tsp pumpkin pie spice
- 2 tbsp honey or maple syrup
- Ice cubes (optional)

Instructions:

1. Blend pumpkin puree, Greek yogurt, almond milk, pumpkin pie spice, honey or maple syrup, and ice cubes until smooth.

Protein-Packed Cheesecake

Ingredients:

- 1 cup low-fat cottage cheese
- 1/2 cup Greek yogurt
- 1/4 cup protein powder (vanilla or your preferred flavor)
- 2 tbsp honey or maple syrup

- 1 tsp vanilla extract
- 1/2 cup fresh berries for topping

Instructions:

1. Blend cottage cheese, Greek yogurt, protein powder, honey or maple syrup, and vanilla extract until smooth.
2. Pour the mixture into individual serving glasses or a single dish.
3. Chill for a couple of hours before topping with fresh berries.

Oatmeal Raisin Energy Bites

Ingredients:

- 1 cup rolled oats
- 1/2 cup raisins
- 1/2 cup almond butter
- 1/4 cup honey or maple syrup
- 1/2 tsp cinnamon
- 1/2 tsp vanilla extract

Instructions:

1. Mix rolled oats, raisins, almond butter, honey or maple syrup, cinnamon, and vanilla extract in a bowl.

2. Roll the mixture into bite-sized energy bites and refrigerate for 30 minutes.

Raspberry Chia Jam

Ingredients:

- 1 cup fresh raspberries
- 2 tbsp chia seeds
- 2 tbsp honey or maple syrup
- 1/2 tsp lemon juice

Instructions:

1. Mash fresh raspberries in a bowl and stir in chia seeds, honey or maple syrup, and lemon juice.

2. Refrigerate for about 2 hours until the jam thickens.

CONCLUSION

In the final chapter of our journey towards a healthier lifestyle through the Macro Diet, we reflect on the remarkable progress you've made and set the stage for continued success. This chapter isn't just about concluding a book; it's about beginning a new chapter in your life.

Reflecting on Your Achievements

Take a moment to acknowledge your accomplishments. You've learned to balance your macronutrients, discovered new recipes, and developed a deeper understanding of how food fuels your body. Celebrate your victories, both big and small.

Maintaining a Healthy Lifestyle

As you move beyond this meal plan, it's crucial to understand that the Macro Diet isn't just a temporary fix; it's a sustainable way of eating. We delve into strategies for incorporating macro-conscious choices into your daily life, ensuring that your newfound health remains a constant companion.

Setting Future Goals

Your health journey is far from over. Chapter 8 helps you set clear, achievable goals for the future. Whether it's further weight management, muscle gain, or simply maintaining your current well-being, we provide guidance on crafting a personalized plan tailored to your aspirations.

Community and Support

Remember, you're not alone in this endeavor. Connect with others who share your goals, seek advice from experts, and build a supportive network. We highlight the importance of community in maintaining motivation and accountability.

In summary, This marks the beginning of a lifelong commitment to your health and well-being. It's not the end; it's a new starting point. Embrace the knowledge you've gained, and continue your journey towards a healthier, happier you.